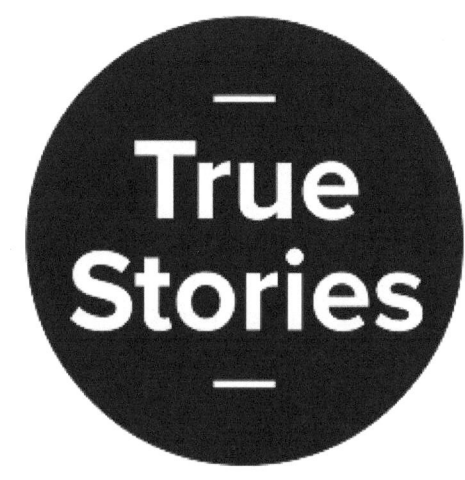

True Stories and True Events

This Book is Dedicated to Each Assistant or Staff Member who has been Tempted, Harass, or Simply made a mistake.

This is good for Nurses as well or really any profession!

NO NAMES SHARED OTHER THAN MINE FOR I SHARE MY STORIES IN HOPES OF SAVING SOMEONE FROM AVOIDING TROUBLE!

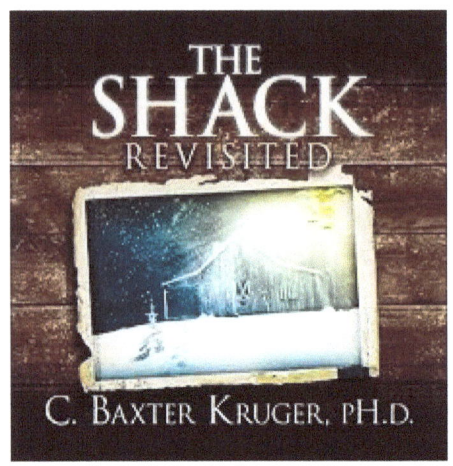

The Shack Dentist

It was my first day at the office and I was so nervous and I remember how one of the Practicing Dentists that was part of the hiring team would ask me questions and one of the questions was did I ever have Government cheese? The office was a place that worked on Underprivileged children and wanted to make sure I could relate to the patients. I of course could relate growing up in a poor home in the inner city of Cleveland Ohio and standing there waiting for the brown box of cheese and boy was it good.

Well getting back to meeting the staff and other Dentist there it seemed pretty nice and I was hoping and praying for the position to be mine. I even sent a fruit basket because it was a chance as the office called it "Getting voted on the Island" How exciting it was to join a big practice if I could.

I did my working Interview of course and landed the position and hey how could I not I was once called the child whisper! I could coach a child into a chair for treatment.

As with any business there will be issues from time to time.The stress level would be up and Good old Doctor would lighten the mood by being funny and so on. Let's call him Dr. Shack because of another reason I will tell later in the story.

Dr. Shack was a ladies man because he had already destroyed one marriage of one of the girls in the office by sleeping with her and the whole office new about it but they insisted on both staying employed there but one worked on one side and the other worked on the other side of the building and the rule was they could not work together. To the blind new assistants because when I was offered the position it could had been given to someone who turns out to be a friend for a season in my life. A very crazy season if I must say. I told the office manager to go ahead and give the job to the new assistant out of school that in fact I felt I could find one more easier but instead she hired us both for my unselfish ways.

I fell in love with the office to the point I called them family some of my readers can relate to this.

Well needless to say me and the other new girl call us Peas and Carrots because we were such good friends but both blind to what would happen as we grew more involved with the office.

Several months went on and everyone was working great together on our team but stress was high and life happens. Doctors come in from home stress out about marriage issues and same with assistants and if happens to be the same day well not a good mix that is for sure but what is worst when a Dentist plans out another notch on his belt which was actually what Dr. Shack was doing. I was just blind to it all. I was going through a bad marriage and I am talking bad from abuse into the frying pan and as I would go into work to take care of others with my bruises beneath my scrubs I was being supported by my work family that I loved so much. I know work is work but you get attached to others you work with. Well the day came that I had enough courage to end the marriage and I attended my local church and just kept praying and because the Dr. Shack new of my belief he decided it was time to try to make another notch on his belt but with my unawareness to what was going on. Let's just say this old city girl was being fooled.

Dr. Shack brought in a book called "The Shack" and he wanted me to read it to help me and I thought how sweet of him. I read it and we discussed the book and it became a bonding moment. I then was asked how are you and your kids doing and that he wanted to meet with me at the end of work at Merchants drive and being from the city I wasn't sure where that would be at so I put in my GPS and agree to meet against my better judgement but he was someone at the office I thought I could trust and was ok with meeting him. When I arrived at the place I noticed it was a liquid store and the better part of town and he was sitting in the car and waved me over. When I got into the car he had already poured not one but 2 glasses of an expensive drink and one I didn't drink but felt I had to at this point for whatever reason I had and I pretended to drink some of it by putting it up to my mouth and acting like I was swallow some but really didn't because well I am against drinking and driving and was not about to get a DUI as we sat there he handed me a Dave Ramsey book and said write down all that you owe and that him and his wife wanted to help me. I was amazed he was going to give me this money to help me and my kids and I even picked up a Thank you card for him and his wife as well as everything I owe written down for his review after all he was going to help me eliminate the debt.

I was on cloud nine out of a bad marriage a few good friends at the time and learning to be free again. Support from work and life couldn't be better.

As time went on he gave the money to me in installments to show I was paying the bills off. Truth be told it was his way of not getting caught with the wife. I realized she had no part in it when I found my Thank you card in the trash with never being taken home for the Mrs. Clue #1

I realized he was after me at this point and my head was turning I was just out of a battered relationship and no self esteem at the time not realizing how much damage was done to me during those years of marriage. I confided in my co-worker who was the one we both got hired at the same time and boy she was a crazy one taught me things like how to walk in high heels and so much and she was my younger and crazy friend who we shared lost of our mother the same year and when she lost her brother I went to his wake for her support we were that close. I told her what was going on and she didn't discourage the whole idea and when others see it is ok you start to think stupid. I started to have a resentful attitude because here I am trying to do right and this man sees me as prey and well being molested as a young girl and how I have been beat up by men all my life I was angry enough to go ahead and do what he wanted because I knew it was pay up time so to speak when he ask me to meet him again this time at a hotel. Not far from the office must be his spot you can say. I am going to be honest, I knew I had to pay up or maybe I would lose my job because he would say something to someone and I couldn't have that. I looked at him with gum in my mouth trying to be a hard ass and said ok let's do this. I laughed at him when he took his pants off for he had boxers briefs on with dam hot dogs on them.

He sat there and cried the pity party and talked about his crooked shoulder as I was waiting to leave since the job was done so to speak and I let him know by shaking his hand afterwards it was just business like I said I was angry. Well

the alcohol was gone the next day and had to get it together to face him and angry that only grew worse within me for another man I looked up to in my life just wanted the same thing.
As I went to my room to set it up for the day of patient's ahead and he comes in with his crossword puzzle and want to talk about it. I shut the door and looked him in the eye and said are you happy you have another notch on your belt? I was even angry at myself for what I did to his wife but figure she knew about all the others and she stayed with him and at the time that was my stupid thinking and the Lord will judge me for this but one of the reasons why I am sharing it so I can help anyone eles from this type of dissaster. Self destruction and being preyed on. I was once told of another assistant who came to his home and sent letters of what he had done. God I wish I could meet her bet she needs healing as well as I had needed. I made sure I came clean with all the appropriate people that it affected and brought it to the light.
I decided to find out more on how often this happens and when I found out more and more I was sickened. He didn't care about race, age, none of it! Total on belt that I am aware of 7!
I explained everything to the office manager but she was to busy trying to turn into Barbie and was losing her lost of true understanding. She did however inform me she knew how he was, Dr. Shack told me once he had stuff on the owner of the practice who was also married

a few times and that his job was secure. So this mistreatment of children were overlooked and as temps came in he would flirt and give things to them as well. When I left and shared with who I needed to share with about how his behavior was it got their attention and truth came out and he was let go only to bring him back a few months later ...Most likely buying more concert tickets for assistants to wheel them in and he most likely has a book club membership Laugh Out Loud, or does he use the same books? Either way I am sure he is still singing I can 7 women on my mind song. I never once received I am sorry from him but believe it or not after signing the papers never speak of this again from the office manager and not to talk to any of my friends at the office since I walked out I thought after a few years no this is my life event that really gave me ptsd that I use it for the greater good and teach every student of mine to be careful out there. I will also share it in my book to use to warn others that it doesn't matter about the Education there are good in bad everywhere and don't be fooled.

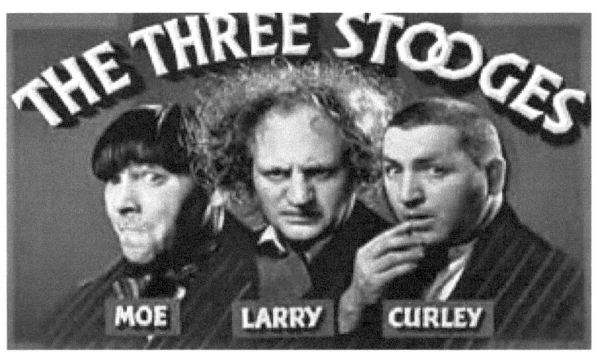

The 3 Stooges Dentist
(Younger Years)

Once there was a Dentist that was married and just had baby #2 and he was a Jewish Dentist not that matters but it stands out because some people hide behind faith and use it to their advantage like the story before.

This Dentist was a General Dentist just opened up a new office. I remember when he asked me to help paint the outside of the office and couldn't help but say yes because I loved my job and my brother was supposed to come help out but never showed up. Thanks brother.The Doctor thank me and walked up behind me and put 50 bucks in my jean shorts and went right out the door.

    I remember clear as day how after that weekend of painting that he came in the next day and said I couldn't stop thinking about you all weekend. Needless to say,I was shocked and amazed by it and it planted a seed that started to grow when it came to the attraction over time and I refused to to have feelings for him but his sense of humor was pretty funny and we worked hard together. I remember he asked me one day in the lab would I sleep with him to go into EFDA school. I was torn up inside over it. I knew if he had any respect for me or his wife he wouldn't ask such a question but this is also coming from a guy who took his head lamp and shine them on my scrub shirt to play.

    Even if I was attracted to him and we had a good relationship as a team even had to go to a meeting and ding dong me drove with him in his car being young and dumb in a shiny fast car and thinking it is all work related. I never said anything to him about what he said previously about couldn't stop thinking about me. I pushed my thoughts out, even though it was a feel good moment that a doctor was interested in me but I knew I shouldn't say yes, I had morals and looked at him crying and said I have to quit my job and worst he just did a crown prep on me and I couldn't get my crown on my tooth so I eventually lost the tooth and forever reminder.

As I was heading for the front door his wife stopped me and asked me why I was crying and why was I leaving. I told her I couldn't say and I quit.

I remember waiting for the bus good old RTA in the big city and having a headache from hell, Like I had no other means to get to work so I found myself desperate for work and took the next job that was offered. I started to lose what I was worth because of needing to pay for bills and just lived. I never had a vacation like most always seem to be a struggle but I decided what I did was way better morally than advancing in my career.

Years later went on and came across the same Dentist and heard through the years he lost his license and had to get them back by volunteering and that him and his beautiful wife were divorce what a shame. Who didn't see that coming because even after I had to show up for my last check and that was hard to do. I remember the new girls in the room with him because I only went to the front office and they both were giggling with him and I could just see his next attempt The Blond or The Red

Head but looking back now knowing how some use it for prey could have been both.

Funny thing ,He had the nerve to ask me for my number and I took his oh yes I did and I gave mine because it was my turn to show him and so sent a few texts since we were both single and dropped it like a hot potato and enjoy doing it.

This is the crazy part I went years traumatized by this thinking EFDA school must be expensive and to find out in some states which was mine there was no need to take the course self study and do the exam that was it. Amazing isn't it so if you can do this, I encourage you to and have the DDS you work for teach you hands on or watch videos and order the materials. It is a win win for the office, your get paid more and more production gets done, just avoid a situation like mine. You will sleep better at night if you do.

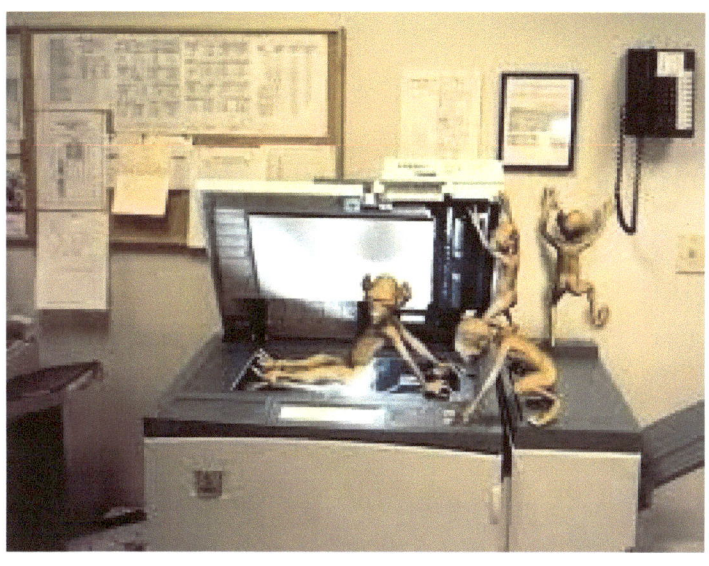

The Copier Room Story
(Right After Dr.Shack Situation)
From one Frying pan into another!

Even at a School It Happened...Some Monkey Business

Once I was teaching at a school that charges students about 17,000 and I made little over 1,500 for the whole month of teaching and the school added stress on the teachers to do homework as well and grading was on my off time. Well on top of that stress but out of the situation in the very first story where the Dr. Shack was out of my daily life. Now I was at a school and things should be much better with the sexual harassment or how I like to call it I wasn't prey no more!

Well I was the Instructor that open up the classroom and help get it ready and I loved preparing places for success if they are doing good that means I did a good job. Well I always had copies to get made for test or homework. I would go into the copier room and always see the second in command in there and we laugh and joke and move on.

Well, she started to come into my classroom when no students were there and would have me look at the photos on her phone just talking as Co-Workers do and one day she said look at my room and this is my bed after we made love. She said a little more but I just went home to my hubby and talked about my day including the strange moment.

The next day I went into work and discovered she was in my room wanting to talk and wanted to invite me and my hubby over and have a cookout. I just didn't feel comfortable with that especially since the day before and especially since my experience with Dr. Shack. One day I went into the copier and the problem is I am a people person, I love to talk and work hard and I see the good in everyone but this day she slapped my butt on the way out! I was in such a shock for a number of reasons one it was another woman and two by a married woman and 3rd at a place that was going to be safe for me. Here we go again.

Well I need more copies oh lucky me and Oh look who is in the room when I opened the door the butt slapper, I get copies made and of course do the small talk so it isn't weird. Then it happened again. SMACK Right on the old bottom! I had it and PTSD came in and said please do not ever do that again! I don't feel comfortable with it. Then went on my way. Needless to say I was then a target and my work was being picked on and my students. I had other issues at the time with the school with racism and yes it does truly still exist. I was not the one subject to it but some of my students were and I once again spoke up and walked out. Once again I left a job that was frustrating me because it just seemed in my career was there any good people left?

Some time later I ran into her with my husband and did the small talk but this time it was out in the open outside with the sun on us. It's hard to explain any of these people I don't hold a grudge maybe because I have a forgiving heart because we all must know how to forgive when others violate us but it seems I just have experience with others getting in my personal space since I was a little girl. I just regret that they had to be that way because they were jobs I loved with or without issues I have always loved this career but it has knocked me a few times as I know it has others from social media and people on my YouTube Channel (Theresa Biggs RDA CDA) Dental Tutor or on my blog https://dentalindex.weebly.com

Double Affair In One Office

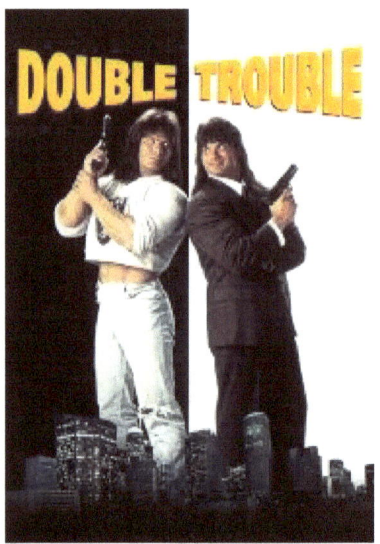

I sit here writing these stories that truly happened in hopes of sharing my personal experience and others have been in this situation other than me and some wanted to get caught up in this situation if you know what I mean.

I will start with one Assistant who had it for one of my bosses and so did the Doctor and it was a shame because I could see them together but no no no not when your married and that was the case here. She shared with me once she shared a kiss at an office party once with him and left it at that. I could see the twinkle in their eyes when they spoke and she worked so hard for him because she really did care for the office. In the meantime you had another assistant there that was crazy for him and for other guys didn't matter if it was a parent of a child or not she would flirt with men.

I use to clean this office and on a Saturday evening before I joined my church and becoming the youngest deacon there I went in to clean the office and there was blood on the floor and cigarette butts as well as beer bottles throughout the office. I called my Employer and said this is unacceptable that I have to clean this up. He said he would take care of it first thing Monday morning but when Monday came along she corner me and said I know you cleaned up and you better not say anything! I was thinking to late and don't care but I just went on my way thinking your going to get yours. Well he didn't do anything instead I moved on because I moved to another state but years later found out she cheated the doctor for years on hours on payroll. He trusted her to write her time down and all I can say is if not faithful to spouse how would you be faithful to anyone else including your employer. It caught up with her and she was let go by work and spouse. Sad because she was beautiful and had it all from home to kids and just destroyed because of an affair and a one night stand and a cheap piece of jewelry.

Don't fall for it! As for the first Assistant she moved as well which she still is happily married and should be because no man or woman should ever come between a spouse no matter how much you think there could be something there, Well there is and that is temptation that most over look and it easy to do unless your are aware of it before hand and you have someone cheering you on to not do somthing stupid but to many times others encourage you to do wrong because we all love a good show and that is where they fall short. If others really care for you they wouldn't encourage such behavior.

      Attraction will happen and if it tempting to and the other party is willing then you know you must walk away because if you are married then even thinking of the other person in a lustful way is just wrong. You must stop that stinkin thinking or better yet. Watch how they are with others and you will lose that feeling because we all know there is turnover in the dental field and the next Assistant could be more than your replacement but an interest. Don't be fooled by the DDS behind the name. They have male parts just like any man but it is not just men since I know first hand woman are doing it as well. I bet their is a male assistant out there wishing he could share how he doesn't like the advancement but must be harder for a male assistant because most men would be like Dude your boss likes you and your not hitting that! Like the movie Horrible bosses which come on if they added that in the movie you know it is a known fact this is happening in the Dental world.

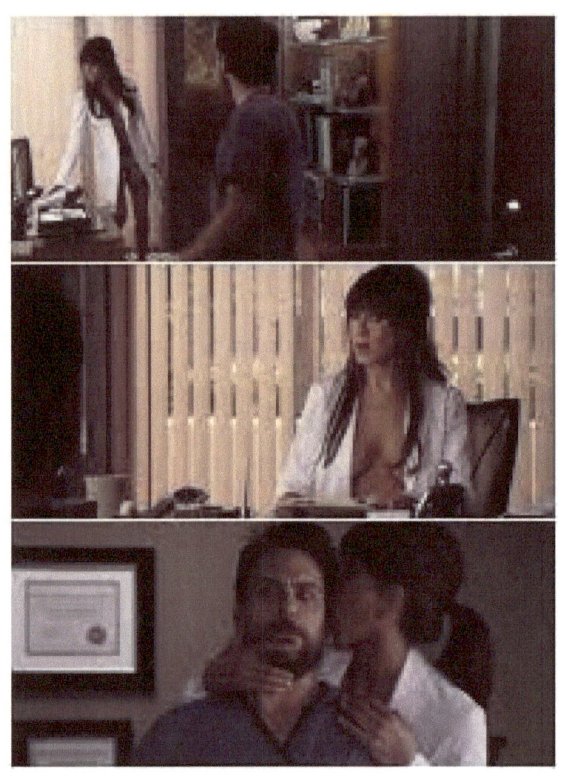

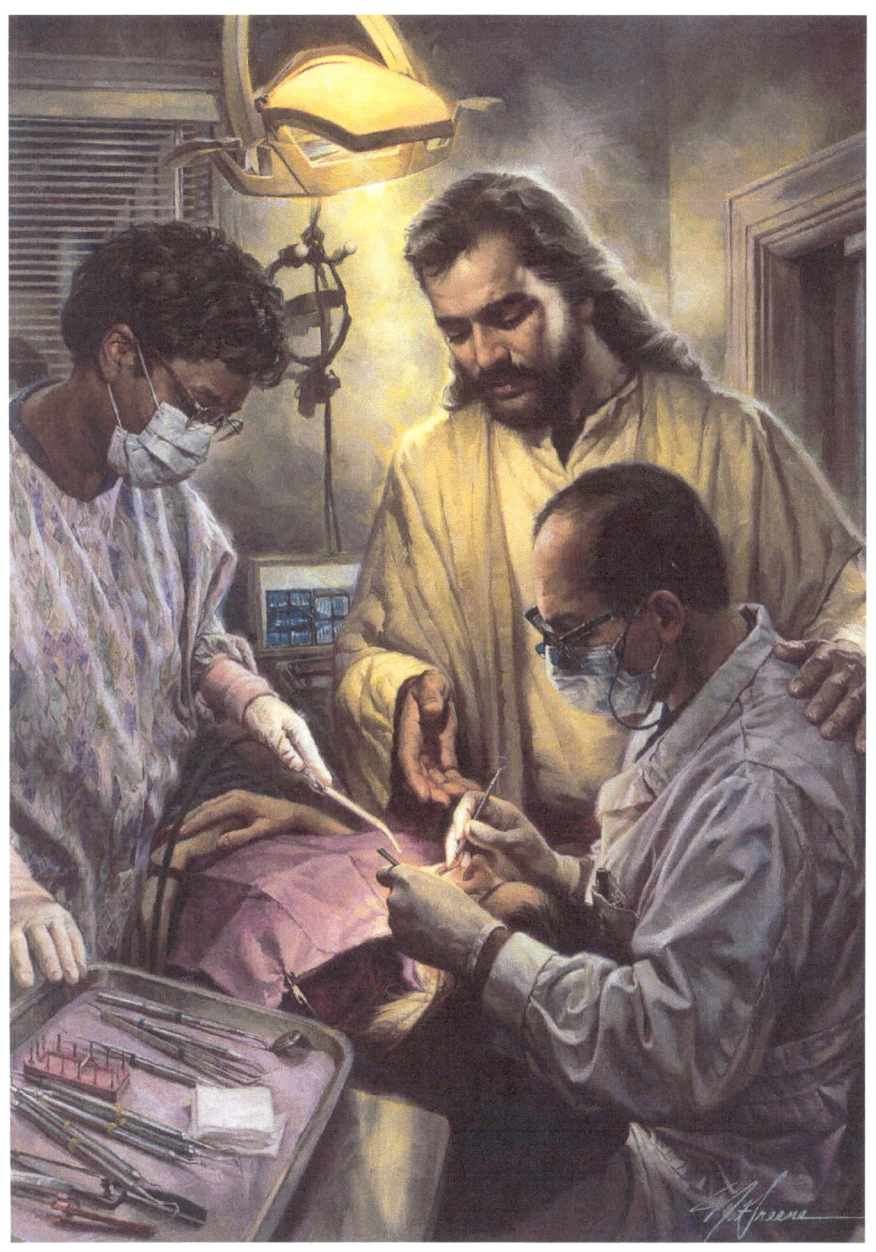

The Christian Dentist

Now another story that I witnessed but didn't realize it till after the blow out. Yes blow out and this is what happened. I was brand new to the State and had faxed my resume prior leaving my hometown before moving I got the yellow pages online and went to Craigslist for my new town that I will be moving to and set up interviews for when I got there. I had a mishap and had not one but two broken elbows with no cast because I was moving out of state and I said my goodbyes at the school I hold dear to my heart because I fell in love with teaching others this career there. Never thought I could do it and others had bets the students but It was meant to be and they students knew I cared. I met the Doctor and yes his wife at the interview because she worked there and once again my blinders were on as well as everyone else's in that office including the beautiful good hearted wife. I had fun at the office and learning how Southern folks are and it was awesome but life change for me once I moved down here found myself with an abusive man and all I knew down here with my son. I didn't have nowhere to go but to deal with it. I went to work with bruises and always hidden but hey I had brand new scrubs on and make and hair done so no one would notice I was being hurt. I felt safe going there because the girls where a joy and loved working with them. I worked with one lady she had a rack on her and she joked about it all the time and I was still walking in faith and learning at that time so I just joked along and the Dentist didn't like laughter in the office but yet looking back now Christ followers should have more peace in their heart and enjoy a laugh or to and I have to share it because his practice was built on being a Christian office and him and his wife would do mission trips. I admired that about them and here I am with this man hurting me and controlling me. Well I always am liked at an office and I always did my work. I guess that's why and one day I wanted to look more like my mother who died when I was 11 and was like a vegetable since age 2. So I dyed it black and boy bad timing to get my nails done and yes it is a no no but this office you could and I wanted to fit in so I got them done and black tips design it was cute but the Dentist said I bother his spirit and that I was looking Goth. WOW the bother my spirit really made me think. Well, I lost it because I won't be spoken to like that well at least when I am not afraid of the person. I left crying because it hurt and plus he told me to go home and dye it back. He said I looked beautiful at any other time. Well I grabbed my purse and when I did the door shut hard on the cabinet and well needless to say I didn't go back and try to get unemployment but in this state it is all up to the Boss but I fought and I knew I wouldn't win but kinda had hopes on the Justice system but he brought two of the assistants with him and they bold faced lied and I got so mad because I could not believe this was happening they were supposed to be Christ followers and you don't lie. Still learning about true Christianity and well we all fail at times and you just don't hold it against anyone. We are tempted by the flesh but we must learn from each others experiences so they don't fall. Well that's my thinking on it. Moving on I left and years later guess what I spoke to one of the ladies from the office that was always super sweet. She told me that after I left a little while later that the Office Manager/Assistant Fill in was having an affair with the boss and that the other lady knew about it! That explain why these two ladies lied and helped him. What a shame because the lady was Married to a Super Bowl Star and the wife to the Dentist was her best friend since they were kids. Amazing how you get validation but also sad to hear of such news for the innocent party and for their marriage. I also realized that one of these ladies filled in for me at another office and I don't know if she knew it was me but hey I left a Thank you note and made all her trays up to be kind. To show forgiveness. Two wrongs don't make a right!

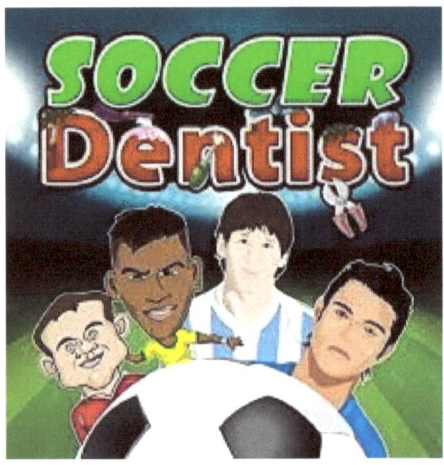

The Soccer Dentist

There was one time when after I had experience all this that I found myself working at an office once again that I loved. The problem was I had prayed while unemployed after school to go ahead God you put me in places of employment to do good and to help make a change and as crazy as this sounds to the non believer it is my belief and I must always give him credit during times he has completely saved me from making horrible mistakes as some have failed but even if you have failed you can make it right and move forward.

Moving on with the story I was hired and within a week I was told of the attraction between the Hygienist and The Doctor. I was like in my head thinking here we go again and thank God I am safe because there was no attraction on our end. You don't want to work for someone you think is eye candy it will never work out.

I started noticing what the other girls where noticing and before I was hired the last assistant that I took her place and I got to know her some through the girls working there and I like her she told me she straight up told the Dentist not to hang out because she talked to him like a brother and told him what he did wrong. Well since she left why worry about the one who complain and keep on doing what you're doing and it seemed to be some flirting going on and you can tell by the body language. You know the Bottom up when leaning on the counter and the Dentist is right there and we all know those rooms are not that small. She even grabbed his phone once and went through it with everyone at the meeting can we say that is a sure clue? I really liked his wife and him and my husband and I made hand crafted wood stuff for him to say thank you for being a good boss and I would still be there but I had no idea he was going to fire two of the ladies working there for a number of reasons and if I was a boss and I knew what he knew I would have sat them down and talked to them. He owed them that because he took away the retirement he couldn't afford and that well just left a bad taste so to speak to the team. Can't blame them but also the action where there and the one girl who had a crush on the Dentist even said from another office where another affair was happening " Well why didn't he pick me" like wow so you see some want that attention. I don't think I could have stayed there and stomach if it was true and that is why he got rid of them? Not for their lack of care for office that was caused by him for taking away the retirement that could have been fixed, especially how long they both worked there for him. I decided after that office as some of my subscribers know on my channel that I couldn't work no more for an office because it just too much of a heart ache for me seeing others lives ruin or even mine own a time or two or at least it felt like it was over.

    I am here! it is never over just sometimes you need time to heal from an office that has done you wrong in any way. As well forgive yourself if you are doing the wrong. You will be amazed how much less stress you feel for forgiving others and yourself.

    -Theresa Biggs RDA, CDA
        Dental Instructor AKA Dental Tutor

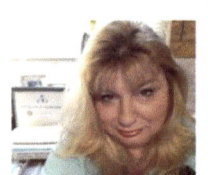

WEBSITES
STUDENTS https://dentalindexjr.com
DENTAL PROFESSIONALS https://dentalindex.com
DENTAL ADVICE https://thedentalgeek.weebly.com

DENTIST WEBSITES CREATOR

TUTORING SERVICE TO ALL DENTAL ASSISTANT STUDENTS/OR ENROLL FOR ONLINE OR TRAVEL TO YOU

RESUME -ORTHODONTIC ASSISTANT.-
RADIOLOGY-DENTAL ASSISTANT-
ADMINISTRATIVE DENTAL ASSISTANT COURSES

PORTABLE DENTAL UNIT FOR PRACTICING SUCTING
"EVERYDAY I AM SUCTIONING"

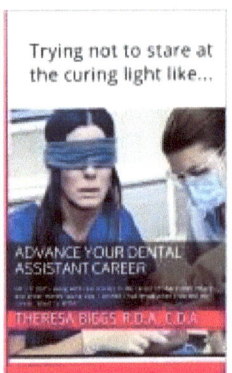
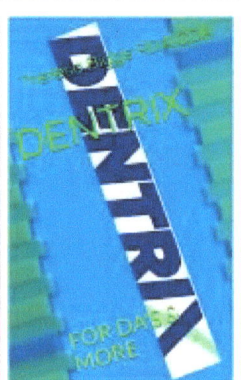
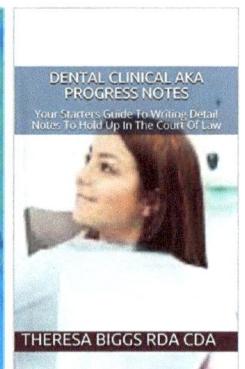

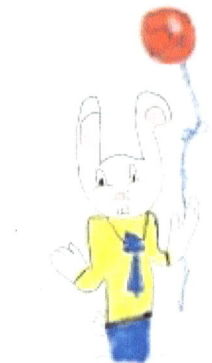

Skipper outsmarted the Bully!

https://www.amazon.com/dp/1091449201/ref=cm_sw_em_r_mt_dp_U_H.wCDbNJSS91Z

By: Theresa Biggs

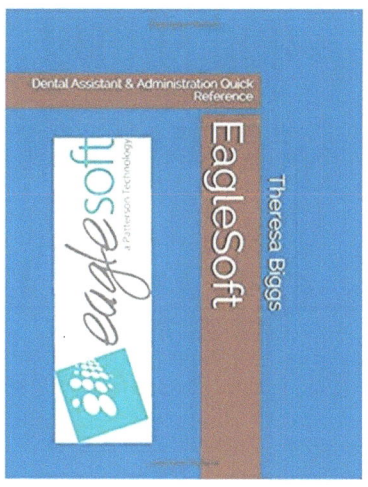

Clinical Notes AKA Progress Notes:
https://amzn.to/317i9jB
Dentrix : https://amzn.to/2Mfg8xm
Eaglesoft: https://amzn.to/2YjtJ9b
Need To Know Book:
https://amzn.to/2YmI7gX
YouTube For Dental Students and News
Youtube channel Dental Index Jr
https://www.youtube.com/channel/UCo6SNeg9l2MlBicGRZxQxcg
The Dental Geek Free Advice Site
https://thedentalgeek.weebly.com
Bigg Faith
https://biggfaith.blogspot.com

GOD FOUND
-some of the-
STRONGEST
WOMEN
and made them
DENTAL ASSISTANTS

Dealing with a toxic work environment can be challenging for both managers and employees.

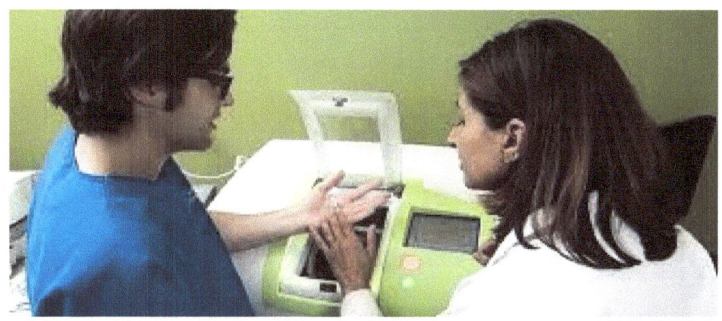

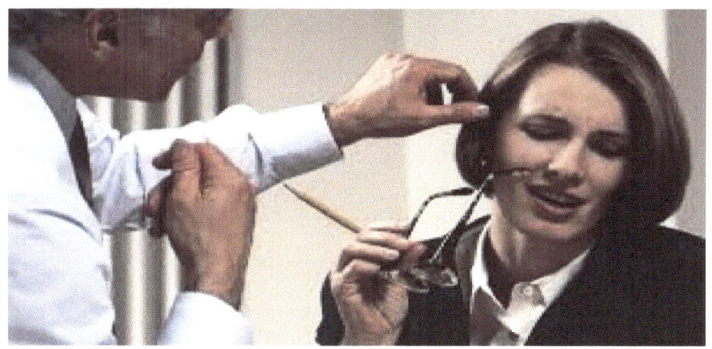

Sometimes it happens when you least expect it!

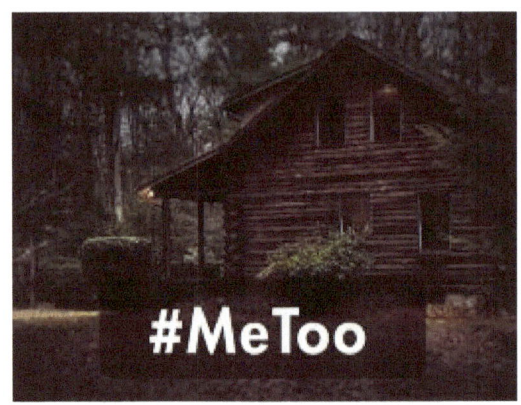

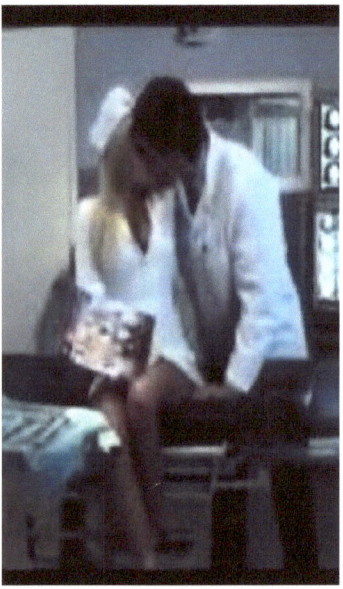

Don't get caught up in a love affair
Not Worth It and try to always have
another person there or door open.

ass-grabbing forced kissing
coercion unwanted sexual emails
stalking unwanted groping
forced touching
pressured sexual activity
sexual harassment
sexual assault cat-calling
unwanted sexual jokes
rape

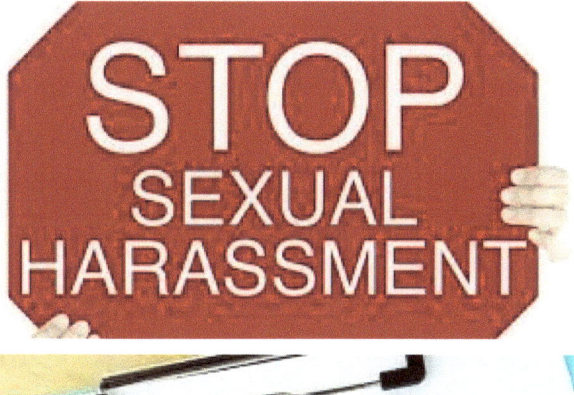

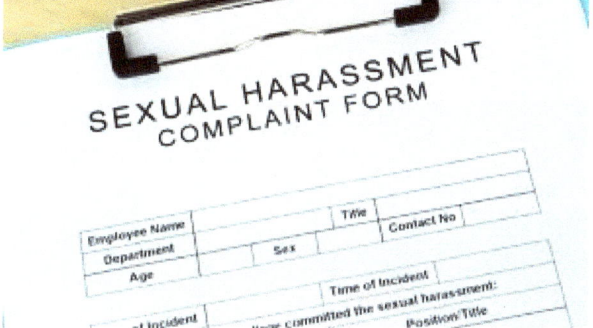

Why do victims stay silent?

societal blaming
embarrassment
humiliation **Fear** trauma family ties
workplace retaliation shame isolation
Who will believe me?
manipulation
reliving the experience financial dependence
further abuse

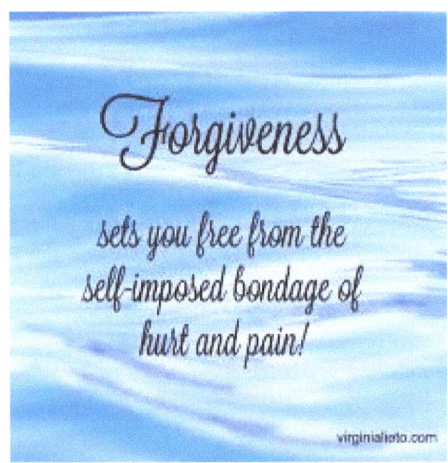

Forgiveness sets you free from the self-imposed bondage of hurt and pain!

virginialieto.com

God forgives you.
Now forgive yourself.

I had to forgive a person who wasn't even sorry...

that's strength.

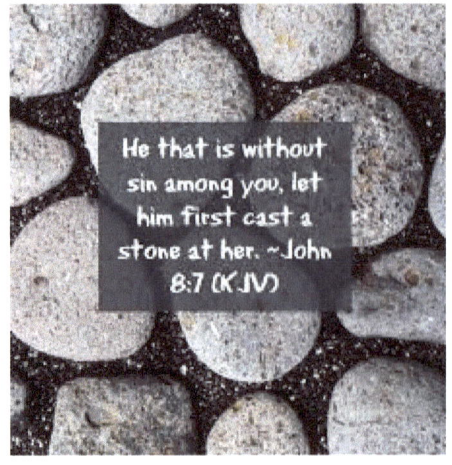

He that is without sin among you, let him first cast a stone at her. ~John 8:7 (KJV)

> "...GOD CAN'T HEAL YOU OF THE PAIN YOU INSIST ON HOLDING."

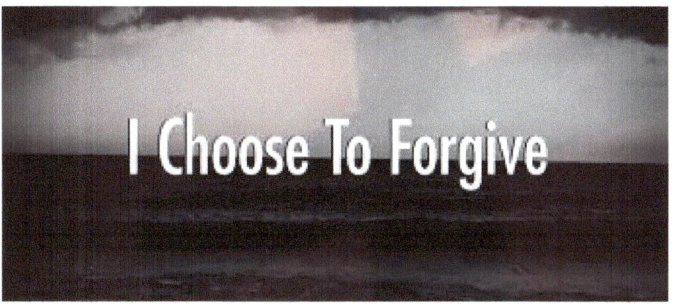

To each Dentist who knows these stories, Especially the ones I was impacted by I Choose To Forgive You.
-Theresa Biggs RDA,CDA Instructor
30 years